THE DUCKLING IN

A Gentle Baby Loss Story

Written by Kara Mangum & Illustrated by Sandy Sanders

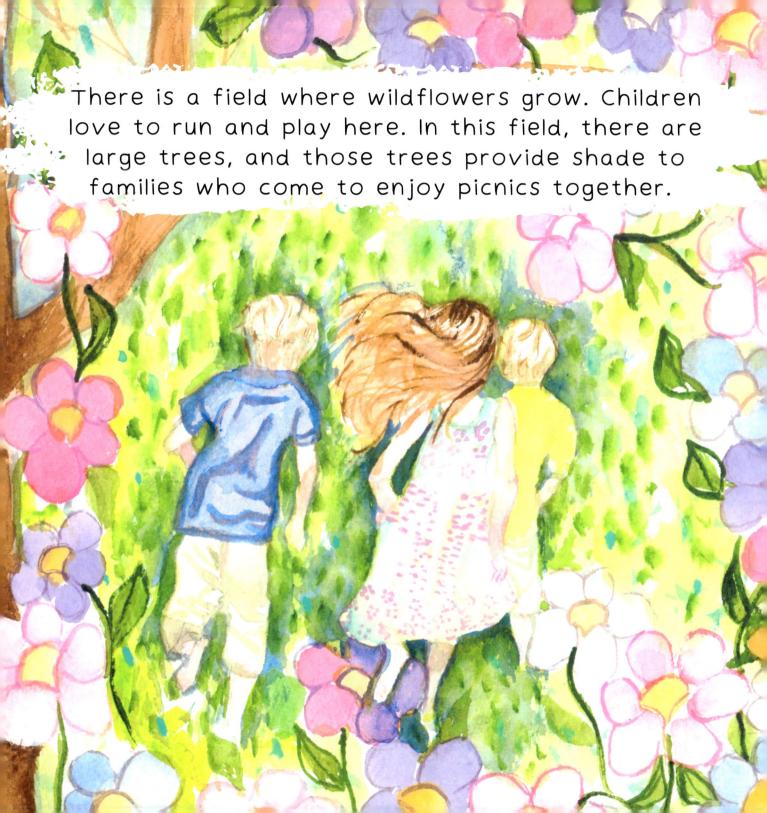

There is a field where wildflowers grow. Children love to run and play here. In this field, there are large trees, and those trees provide shade to families who come to enjoy picnics together.

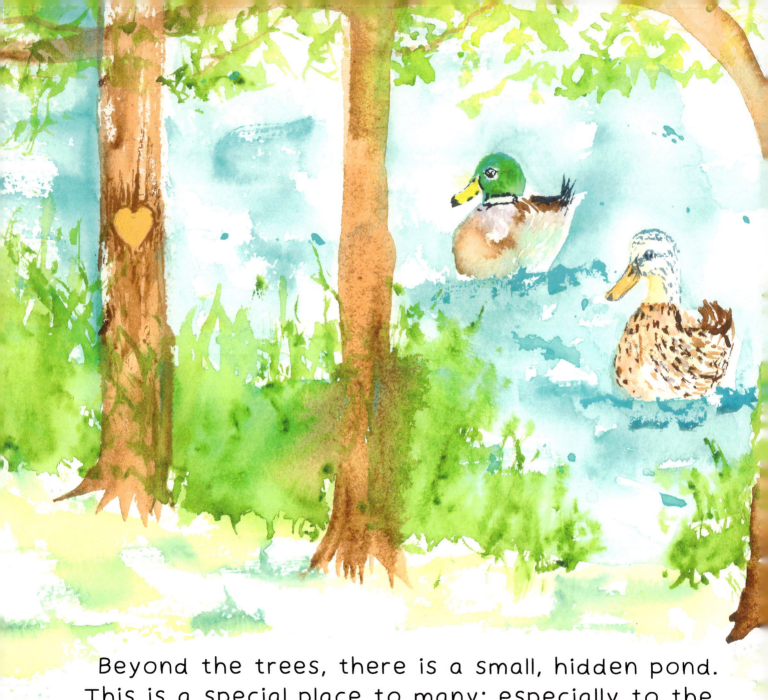

Beyond the trees, there is a small, hidden pond. This is a special place to many; especially to the animals who live here. This is the home to Mama Duck and Daddy Duck.

To all families who know what it is like to carry the memory of their babies in their hearts.

Mama and Daddy Duck are working diligently to build a new comfy nest. They are creating a nest because Mama Duck needs a safe and quiet place to lay her brand-new egg.

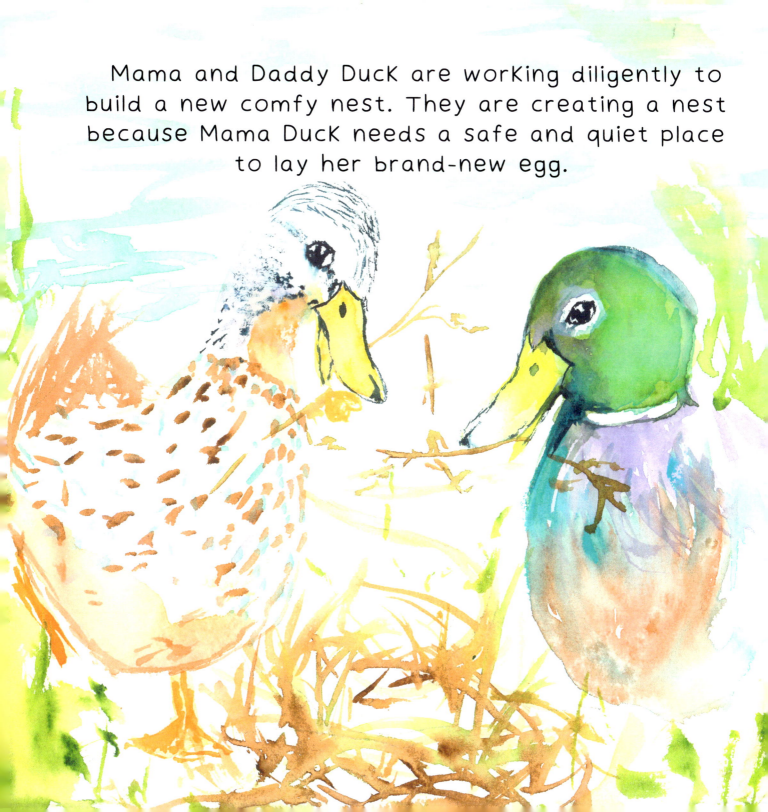

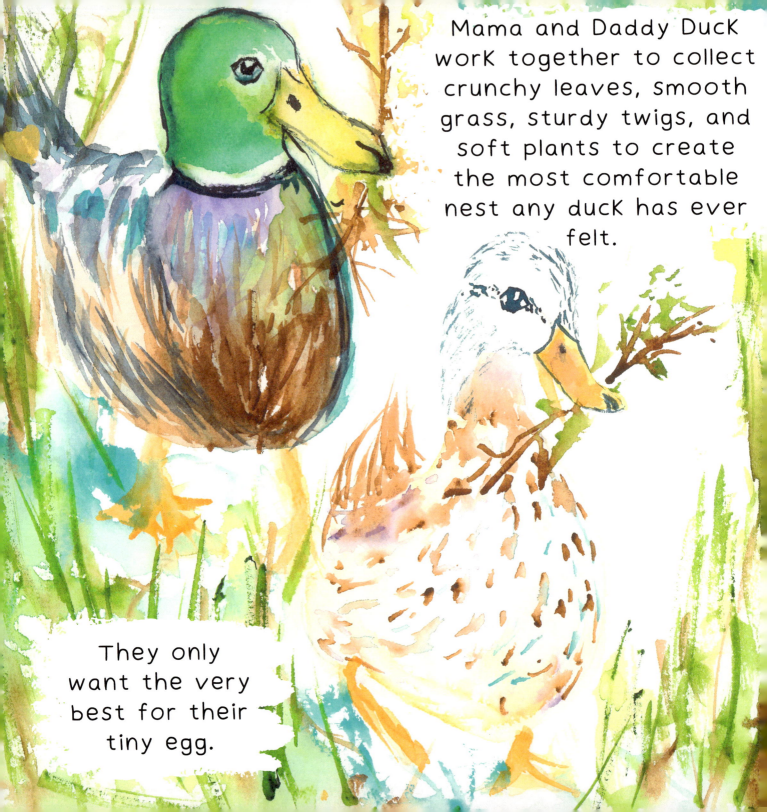

Mama and Daddy Duck work together to collect crunchy leaves, smooth grass, sturdy twigs, and soft plants to create the most comfortable nest any duck has ever felt.

They only want the very best for their tiny egg.

Once Daddy Duck placed the finishing touches on the nest, Mama Duck knew it was time to lay her shiny new egg.

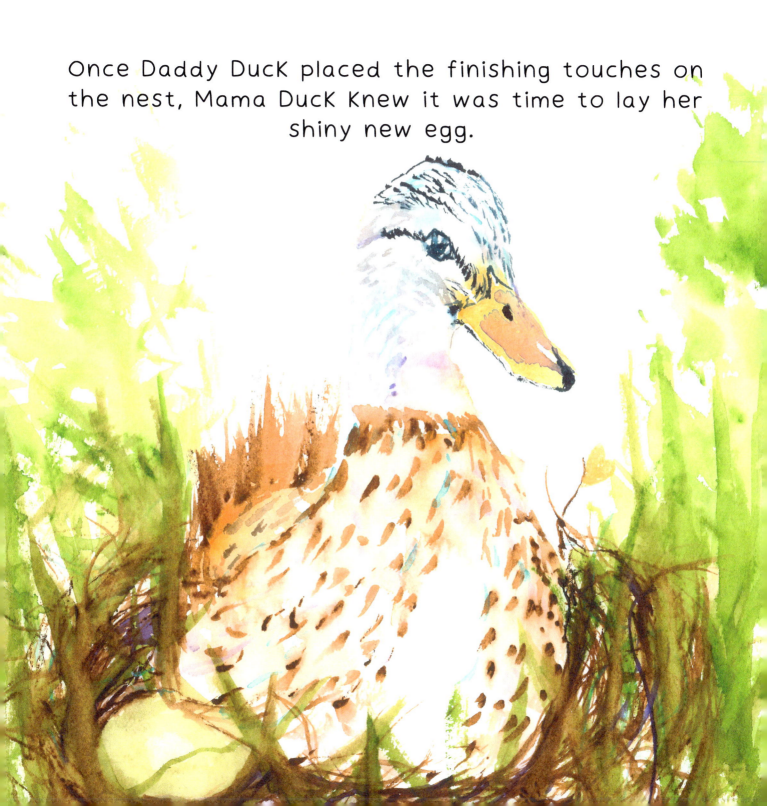

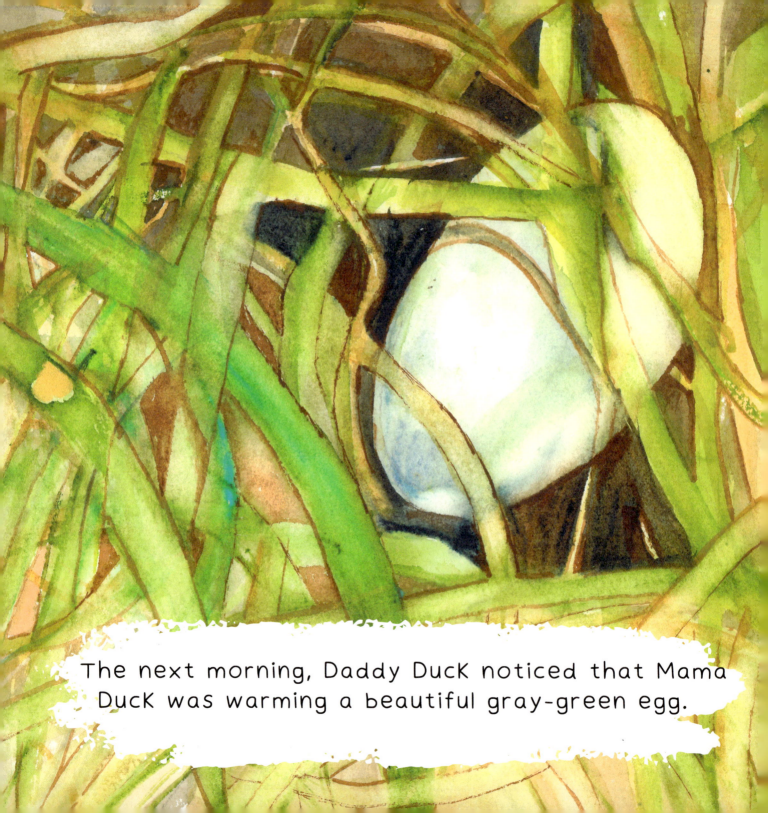

The next morning, Daddy Duck noticed that Mama Duck was warming a beautiful gray-green egg.

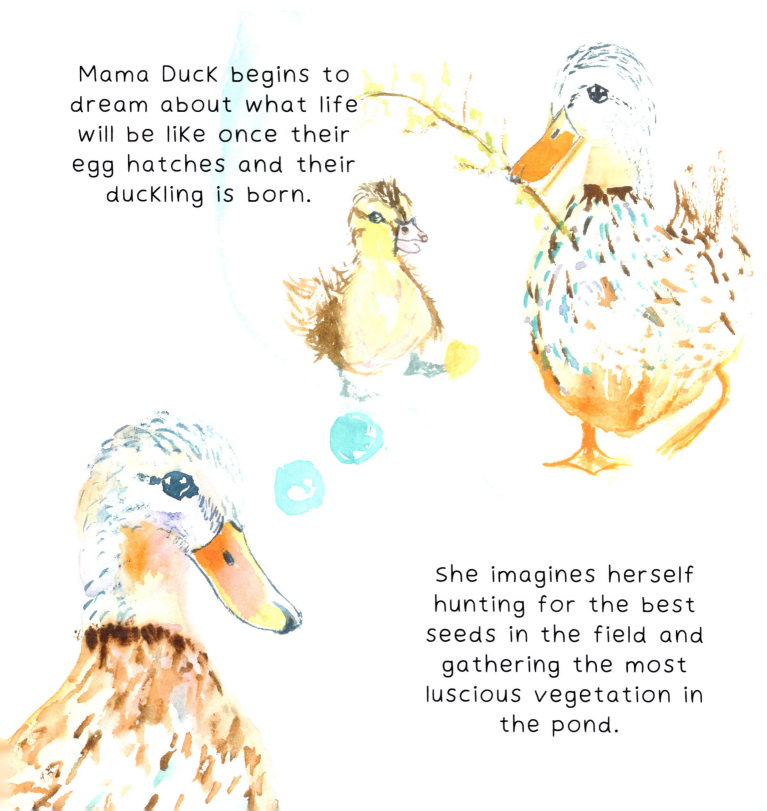

Mama Duck begins to dream about what life will be like once their egg hatches and their duckling is born.

She imagines herself hunting for the best seeds in the field and gathering the most luscious vegetation in the pond.

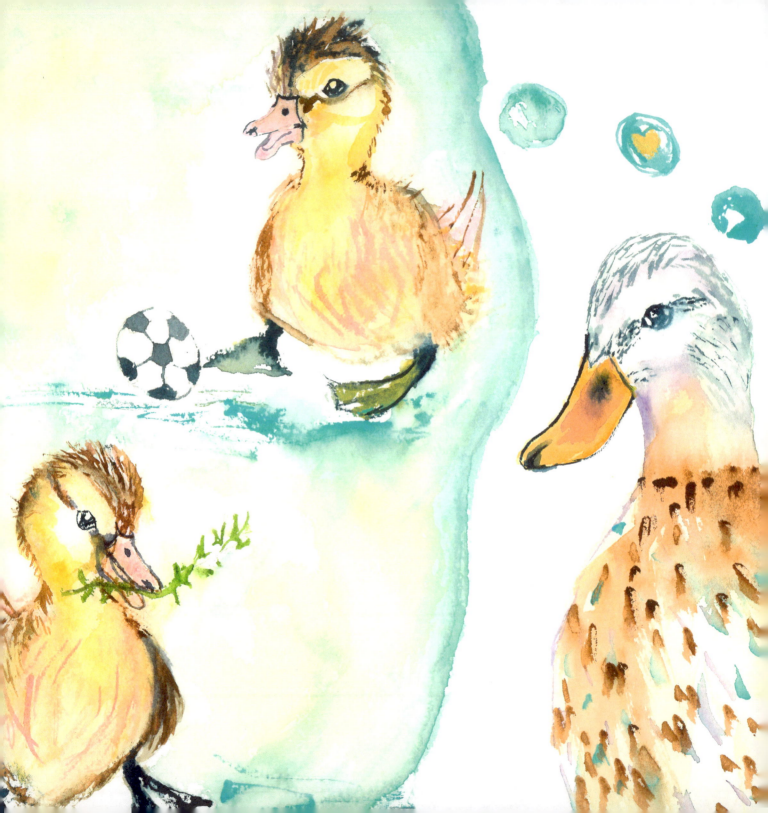

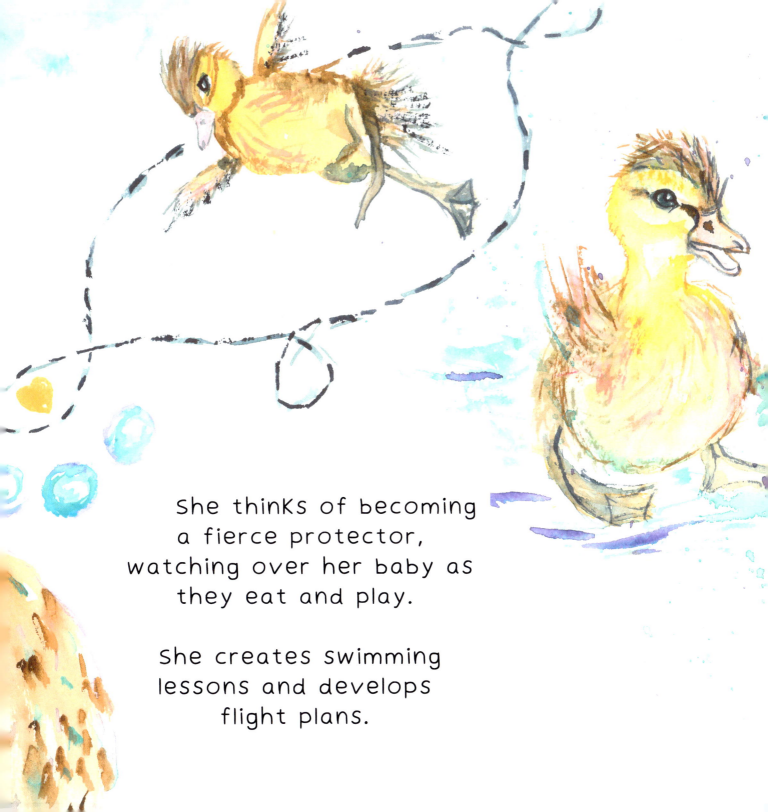

She thinks of becoming
a fierce protector,
watching over her baby as
they eat and play.

She creates swimming
lessons and develops
flight plans.

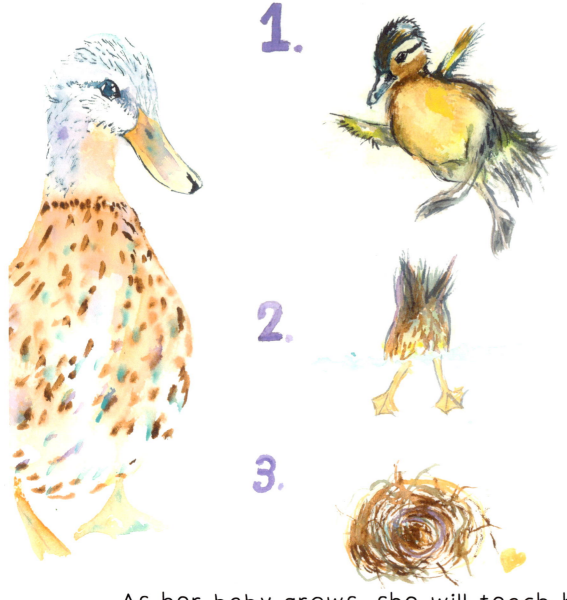

1.

2.

3.

As her baby grows, she will teach her little
duckling how to fly, how to hunt, and even how
to build their own nest one day. She Knows life
with her duckling will be filled with the greatest
of love and the most wonderful adventures.

Mama and Daddy Duck become so excited as they patiently wait for the little egg to hatch.

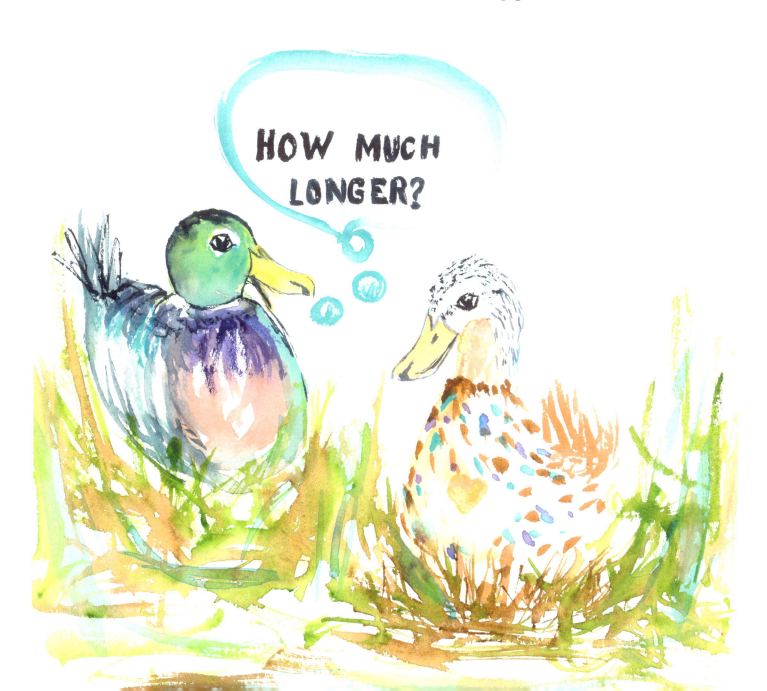

As they wait, they begin to talk about this little duckling. Will the duckling be a boy or a girl? Will their name be Daisy, Jemima, Huey, or Little Quakers? Oh, how could they choose? There are so many great names. How could they possibly select the perfect one?

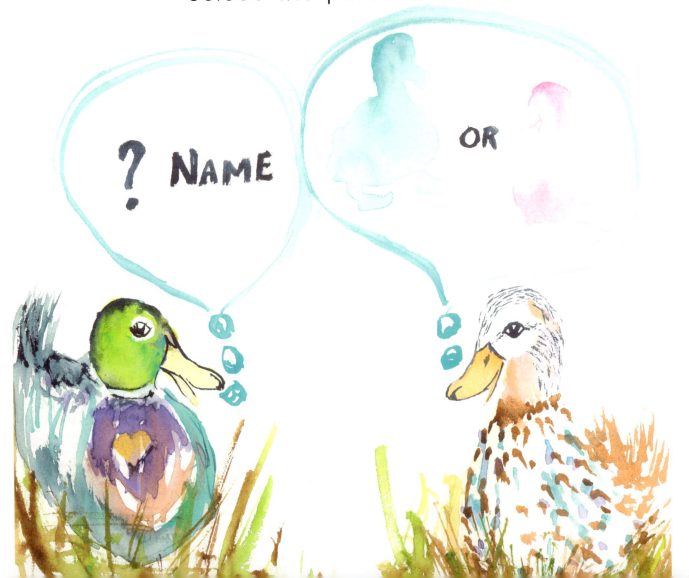

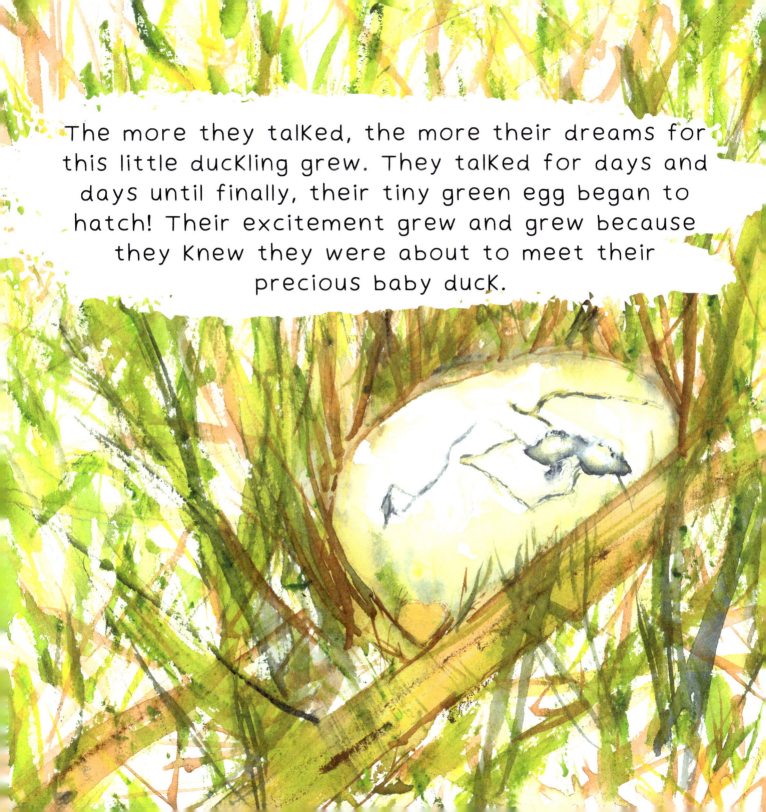

The more they talked, the more their dreams for this little duckling grew. They talked for days and days until finally, their tiny green egg began to hatch! Their excitement grew and grew because they knew they were about to meet their precious baby duck.

But as the egg began to crack and open wide, they realized their baby duckling wasn't inside.

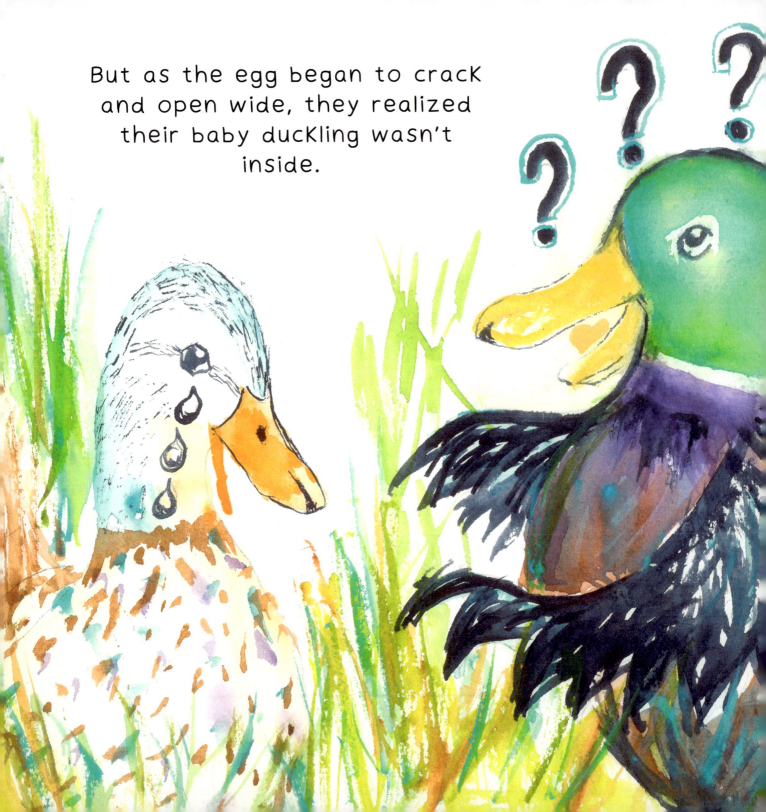

The egg was empty. Daddy Duck did not understand. Mama Duck began to cry. How could this happen? Why did this happen?

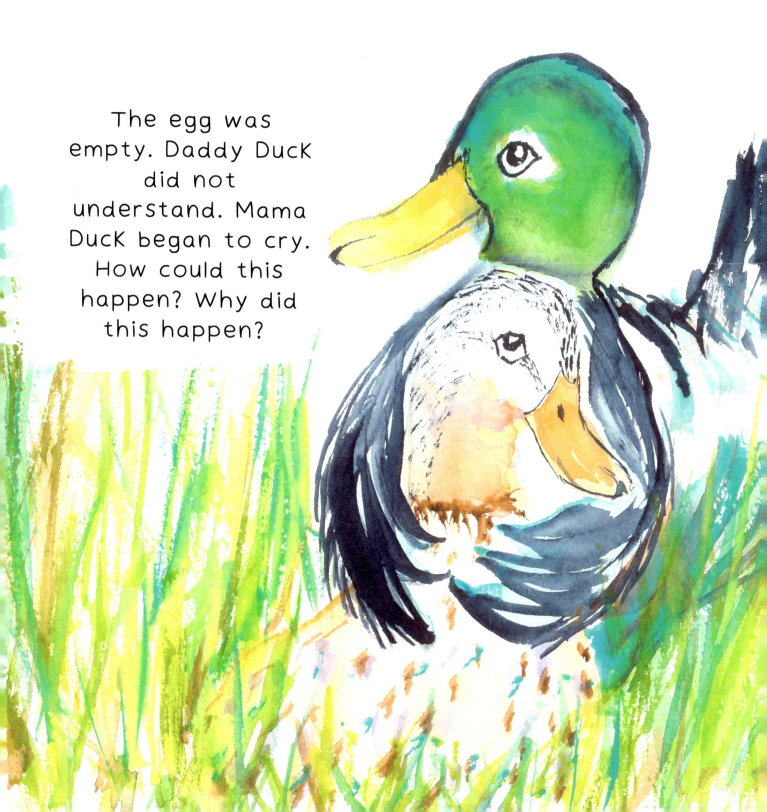

There were so many questions and those questions would be left without answers. Mama and Daddy Duck were devastated by this news. It took some time to heal and for their tears to be dried. They would always remember their shiny green egg and the little life they thought it would bring.

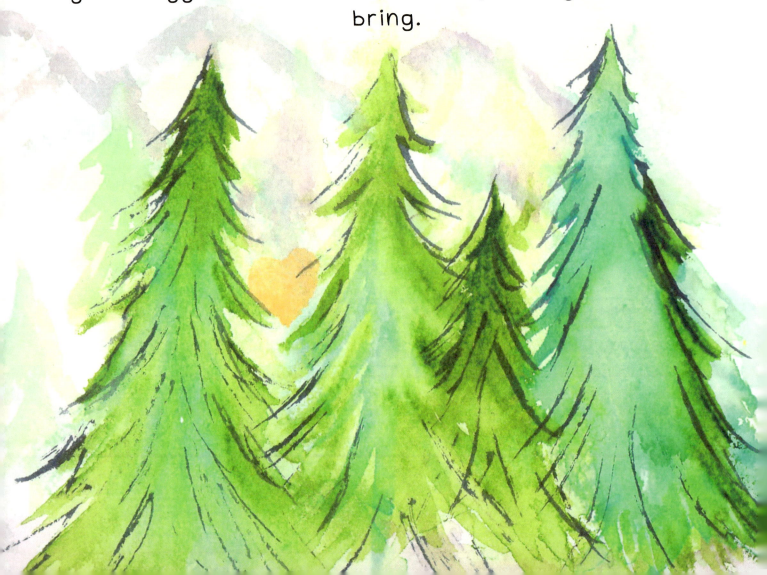

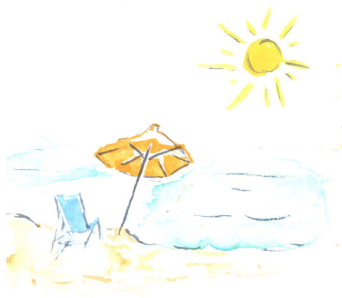

As the seasons began to change, from summer to autumn, and then to winter, they remained hopeful for the opportunities that next spring would bring.

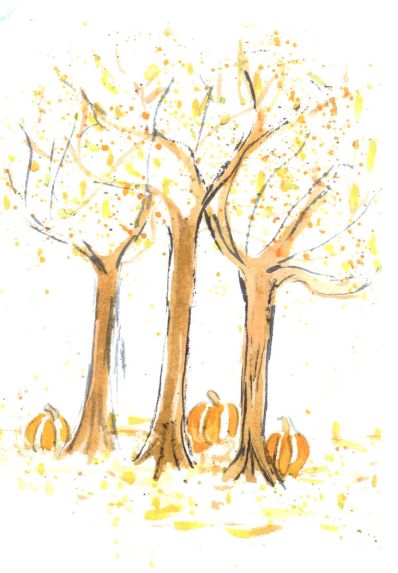

Mama and Daddy Duck think about their little duckling each day. What would their days have been like with their baby swimming by their side?

Now, Mama and Daddy Duck work to honor their duckling. They help other animals around the pond, and in the field, as they remember their tiny egg and the baby duck that was supposed to be. There will always be a special place in their hearts for their precious duckling. This will remain true both now and forever.

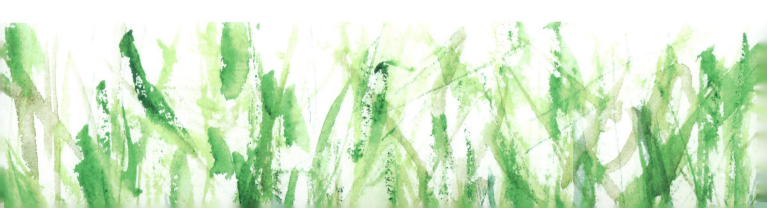

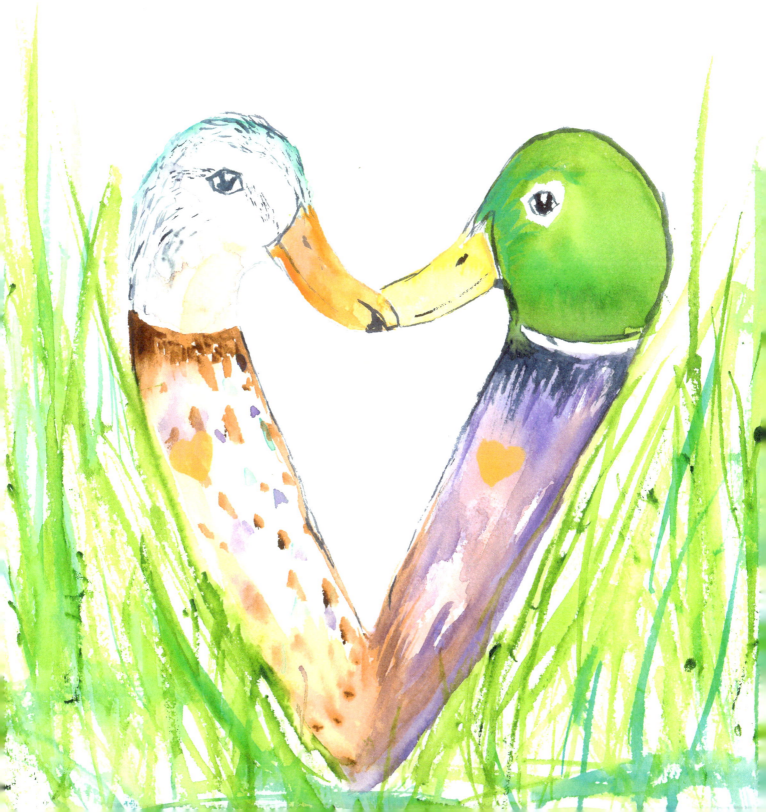

A Message from the Author

Dear Reader, I hope this book serves as a valuable tool and helps you explain the difficult process of pregnancy loss to a young child. I intended this story to be gentle so it would be appropriate to use for a range of ages. The empty egg in this story is symbolic of the death of our babies. This is not intended to diminish the physical existence of our babies but instead allows the parent to discuss what is developmentally appropriate for their children.

For those of us who have experienced a pregnancy or infant loss, we know what it means to carry the memory of our baby within our hearts. Some of us had the opportunity to hold our babies in our arms, while others did not. Our babies will always have a special place within our hearts. It is through our hearts that the memory of our babies live on.

Can you find the golden hearts?

There are golden hearts placed within the illustrations, symbolizing the memory of our babies. Our babies are precious, they matter, and they will never be forgotten. I encourage you to search the pages for golden hearts with your children. Use them as a way to connect on a deeper level. Study the illustrations together and discuss the feelings and emotions each of you are experiencing. Make sure to take time to listen and understand what your child is going through. Remember, each of us grieves differently. We grieve in our own way and in our own time. I hope you enjoy searching for hearts together. I hope you are able to have productive discussions and are able to support one another while each of you grieve. I hope you then work together to create your own way to honor and remember your baby or babies.

Always remember, you are loved, you are prayed for, and you are not alone.
With Love, Kara

Dear Reader,

The journey of grief can be isolating and unpredictable. Everyone will experience grief and yet, so often, we feel alone and as though our situation of loss is unique. It is so important that we are patient with ourselves when we walk the path of darkness, because finding the light can seem impossible. But I believe that every dark Good Friday ends in a bright Easter morning.

Loss is a very important part of life and needs to be courageously embraced so healing can transform us. The greatest Biblical miracle was performed at the grave by our Almighty God so we can rest in His comfort, sovereignty, and promise of hope that no loss is too great to go unanswered by God.

Say "Yes!" to the path of grace and mercy that has your name on it as you walk hand-in-hand with your Savior in the new places of understanding His love for you. God has healing, light, and hope for you as you trust Him to carry your broken heart. He doesn't just want you to survive grief, He wants you to be filled with a new JOY!

You are loved, you are not alone, and you are known.
"Even the darkness will not be dark to you; the night will shine like the day, for darkness is as light to you."
~ Psalm 139:12
~ **Linda Znachko Founder of: He Knows Your Name Ministry** – heknowsyourname.org Author of: "He Knows Your Name – How One Abandoned Baby Inspired Me To Say Yes To God"

Our Hearts Align is a 501(c)3 nonprofit organization dedicated to serving families who have experienced pregnancy loss and early infant loss. We provide care packages to families and connect them with resources that meet their specific needs.

Throughout the different stages of pregnancy loss, families often feel alone and have many questions. It is our mission to be a support system. To provide you with resources to help you grieve and honor your baby. We also want to help you feel comforted and to assure you that you are not alone.

Learn more about Our Hearts Align:
www.ourheartsalign.org
Facebook & Instagram: Our Hearts Align

To connect with Kara Mangum:
www.passioninthepurpose.com
Facebook/Instagram & YouTube: Passion in the Purpose

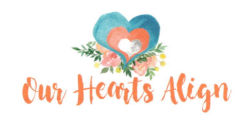

About the Author:

Kara Mangum is the founder of Our Hearts Align, a nonprofit organization dedicated to serving families who experience pregnancy loss. She graduated from the University of Florida with a Master of Education degree. She taught in a classroom setting for four years and now enjoys sharing educational resources on her blog, Passion in the Purpose. Kara is from North Central Florida; where she currently resides with her husband and three daughters. She experienced her own pregnancy loss in 2013 and has since been working to create new resources to help support families during miscarriage, stillbirth, or early infant loss.

About the Illustrator:

Sandy Sanders is a Florida artist who is inspired by life at the beach. The colors of the beach, the reflection of the light, and all of the sea creatures and birds inspire many of her themes and color palettes. She also enjoys painting other animals and pets. Painting is her third career. Previously, she worked as a pediatric nurse and a full time mom. Now,she is a watercolor artist. Her work is on display at Gallery B, a fine art gallery, located in Ocala, FL.

A note from Sandy: Illustrating this book has been a special project for me. I lost a baby at 25 weeks many years ago. That experience was very difficult. As I was creating the illustrations for this book, many emotions came flooding back. I hope this book will help families to process their grief in loss.

About the Formatter

Colleen Reagan Noon of the Wise Women Book Collective is a publishing strategist and focuses on helping publish books that support and empower women. Colleen had two miscarriages before the birth of her two boys. This experience is part of what ignited her passion for women's health and healing.

Made in the USA
Columbia, SC
15 January 2025

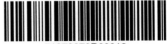

51878279R00018